Walking in Fear...

How I was introduced to my Brain Aneurysms

by
Susan M. James

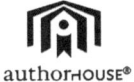

authorHOUSE®

AuthorHouse™
1663 Liberty Drive, Suite 200
Bloomington, IN 47403
www.authorhouse.com
Phone: 1-800-839-8640

First published by AuthorHouse 3/17/2008

ISBN: 978-1-4343-6456-2 (sc)

Library of Congress Control Number: 2008900945

Printed in the United States of America
Bloomington, Indiana

This book is printed on acid-free paper.

THANK YOU

To my loving and supportive husband, Lancelot, whose altruism was paramount to my recovery.

To my daughters, Christine and Cheyanne; I could not tell you initially what was going on, because I did not understand it and I did not want to scare you.

To Gina; I feel that your prayer was the turning point in my survival. I am eternally grateful to you and deeply sorry about your dad.

To Tidewater Volleyball Association; your quick response during my moment of crisis is credited for my survival.

To Mom; your prayers and multiple nights spent with me in the hospital will never be forgotten. Dad, your prayers and encouragement inspired me to keep strong.

To Dr. Dillon at Sentara Virginia Beach General Hospital, and Dr. Agola at Sentara Norfolk General Hospital, as well as all the wonderful nurses in the intensive care units; your expeditious care and concern sustained my life.

To Dr. Rodrigue, Nurse Bowes, and Dr. Rivet at Naval Hospital, Portsmouth, Virginia; Dr. Armonda and Nurse Durand at National Naval Medical Center, Bethesda, Maryland; and all those in conjunction with the intensive care unit. God has blessed you all with the knowledge and skill to care for people like me. Thank you also to Dr. Davis, Sewell's Point, Norfolk.

To my sister-in-law, Althea (Viveen), and my brother-in-law, Clarence; we are eternally grateful to the both of you.

To my sisters, Donnette and Vilma; Aunt Hope; my brothers, Horace and Ricky; my friend Jackie; and my niece, Kisah.

To my friends and coworkers; your prayers and support inspired me to get well. Specific recognition goes out to Tina Nelson; Tammy Hartlen; Lydia Fontanez; Mrs. Benns, ITC (Ret.); Delisa Jones (Magwood); ET2 McNutt; IT1 Battle; YN1 Wood; ITCM Maynard; LT Avitto; IT2 Gwen; and Mrs. B. Wilson.

Annette, although we never met in person, you inspired me!

PRELUDE

Do you ever walk around looking into the faces of individuals you meet, wondering if they are ill but unaware? Well, that's what I started doing after my brush with death.

As an athlete, I play multiple sports, including racquetball, tennis, softball, and the sport I am most passionate about—volleyball. As an active-duty sailor for over twenty-one years, I am required to stay physically fit, so I had incorporated some rigorous aerobic classes into my schedule twice a week in addition to my other physical activities to keep in shape. I kept up with my annual medical examinations and checkups, and I even got my shots as needed. Headaches are something I never suffered from. I have no idea what a migraine feels like. Seizures are conditions I had witnessed in others, and I found them spellbinding.

Sinus pressure in my head is something I had become accustomed to over a few years. When my youngest daughter was born, my family and I decided to travel to Florida every two years to visit relatives, and I eventually noticed a pattern of illness every time I arrived in Miami, as well as throughout certain seasons in my home state. One significant and severe episode I remember is my being diagnosed with vertigo. Shortly after arriving in Miami and checking in at the hotel, I started becoming nauseated. I eventually vomited, and then I noticed that I could no longer sit in an upright position. Sitting upright made me feel like I was being held upside-down and the blood was rushing into my head. After several attempts at sitting up, I decided just to lie down for the duration of the illness. Later that night, my condition worsened and my family decided to rush me to the emergency room. The trip to the hospital was dangerous, because someone tried to run us off the road. My husband swerved to protect us, and we arrived safely. I was unaware of what had transpired and was becoming more ill because of the swerving of the vehicle. We eventually arrived at the hospital, and within minutes, I was seen. After a brief discussion with the doctor about what was happening to me, he ordered a magnetic resonance imagery (MRI). The results of the exam showed that I had a severe sinus infection, and he also diagnosed me with vertigo. Prior to that diagnosis, the only people I had ever heard of having vertigo were pilots. This was my first diagnosis of sinus issues and vertigo, and I was given medication to combat the condition. About four or five days later, I had some reprieve from the condition and was able to function properly and head home.

Two years later, I woke up one morning and was not able to walk straight. I was leaning to the left on my way to the bathroom. I thought that I had either really lost my mind that morning, or that something major was going on. The condition persisted, so I opted to see my doctor that morning. My doctor diagnosed me with another case of vertigo and suggested that if faced with the same scenario, I should do the opposite of what was happening to me to offset the condition. At some point during the day, the condition dissipated.

Throughout the years, I continued to battle with sinus pressure by taking medication that relieved it. The over-the-counter medication helped almost instantaneously, but it also became a way of life. I eventually requested a MRI through my primary care physician to ensure I did not have a brain tumor that was escalating. The results of that examination indicated that all was fine, so I kept on with what I knew worked whenever I had a sinus problem.

MY CLOSE CALL

Wednesday, November 30, 2005, was a life-changing evening for me. My day was filled with my normal routine of going to work, coming home, bonding with my family, preparing dinner, and heading to volleyball for the initial day of our playoffs.

On this particular day, all was well; I didn't even have the sniffles. I had just told my teammates that I would be playing with a minor handicap. I had been suffering from pain in my shoulder whenever I played volleyball, and I had found out earlier that day that my rotator cup was injured and needed therapy. With that in mind, I had to minimize my use of overhand movements. We decided that I would be substituted in instead of starting, because there were six of us playing four-on-four volleyball.

The game began around 7:15 p.m. and we lost the first game. I was substituted in for the second game, and it was a close game. I consecutively served underhand and got the team a few points, which placed us in the lead. I remember that as soon as we were in the defensive position, I was getting ready to receive a ball, but

I started feeling funny. I felt something very cold in my head. It was the equivalent of very cold water on a dry, hot day. The cold fluid ran from fore to aft and from side to side. Shortly after that, things started moving in slow motion, and I remember saying, "Wow!" I was about to tap my teammate to let her know that I did not feel well, and I was concerned that I was having a heart attack even though the problem I felt was in my head. That was all I remembered until I woke up in an ambulance.

I was lying on my side in the ambulance, completely strapped to the transporter bed, vomiting, and suffering from pain in my abdomen and my head. The pain in my stomach was due to the abdominal straps supporting me. The pain in my head was the most profound and excruciating pain I had ever felt in my life. It was worse than childbirth pains. I probably would have answered yes to decapitation if it was offered. I would have done anything to stop the pain! I remember speaking to the emergency medical technicians like I was a two year old. That was the only intelligent way I was able to communicate. I kept complaining about the pain in my stomach and the aggravating pain in my head. My words were, "pain in head, pain in stomach," and I continually vomited. I heard a very comforting voice while traveling to the hospital. There was a Navy Chief in the ambulance who said, "I heard she's a Navy Senior Chief; I'm a Navy Chief, so she's in good hands." Those words were very comforting to me, and they served as my solace in between the pain. I had no idea who the attendants were or what they looked like; I just knew that I was being cared for on my way to the hospital. I was very appreciative as I drifted in and out of consciousness and awareness.

I repeated the words regarding my pain quite a few times before I reached the Sentara Virginia Beach General Hospital. The ride in the ambulance was turbulent—not because the driver did anything erratic, but because the ambulance was susceptible to every blemish on the road.

A short while later, I was awakened, and I saw my husband at the hospital. I needed to use the bathroom and insisted that I be taken immediately. My husband wheeled me to the bathroom and I took care of my business. In retrospect, I don't remember having an excruciating headache at that moment; perhaps I had been given something in the ambulance or in the hospital to reduce my pain. My husband insisted we leave the bathroom hurriedly to resume my care, but I took my time until I was finished. At that point I still did not realize the magnitude of what had happened to me. My husband later told me that he thought I would be okay because I was communicating with him from the time he arrived at the hospital.

Once I was back in the hospital bed, various conversations were going on around me and questions were being asked of my husband by the hospital attendants. My knee pads, underwear, and sweatpants were being removed, and my husband told the attendants I also had knee braces on. I also recall my favorite black T-shirt being cut off of me while drifting in and out of sleep. I thought to myself, *They are cutting off my favorite black shirt; can't they just take it off?*

As the night continued, I drifted in and out of awareness and was told of various exams they would be conducting. I eventually drifted off to sleep. The next day, I became fully conscious of what was going on. I was placed in the intensive care unit (ICU), and I met some wonderful doctors and nurses. My doctor, a neurosurgeon, was very tall and had a kind and caring face. He told me about my brain aneurysm rupture.

Apparently my brain aneurysm had hemorrhaged, which was the culprit behind what had happened to me on the volleyball court. The neurosurgeon stated that I was very lucky, because after the aneurysm ruptured, it resealed itself. That was the first time that I recalled hearing the word *aneurysm*. The magnitude of my medical condition still had not fully sunk in, nor did I realize just how significant it was. My condition was referred to as a subarachnoid hemorrhage located in the distal anterior cerebral circulation. I was also diagnosed with two other aneurysms as well, both located in the intracranial circulation, one on the left side of my head and one on the right. The one on the left was larger than the one on my right.

Several times throughout the following eight days and nights while laying in the in the Virginia Beach Hospital, I was continuously medicated and asked to do various motor skill examinations to ensure that I was coherent and that my faculties were functioning. The doctors and nurses checked my eyes and my medications continuously. I had to raise my hands and legs and answer several questions about such things as my name, my whereabouts, what year it was, the name of the president, etc. I continuously passed those examinations successfully and would sometimes go through the motions before the doctors and nurses would ask. I started experiencing twitching in my arms, but I did not know what it was or why it was happening. I did not discuss it with the doctor; I just knew it was unusual for me and that it was annoying. Each time my arm twitched, I would slap the area and it would subside. Eventually it stopped. Later on I learned that twitching was a result of my condition.

One very poignant memory I have is of the very concerned, puzzling, yet curious stares the doctors gave me whenever they visited me. They never shared what was truly going in their minds, but as a perceptive person, I realized that I was being looked upon as a miracle.

SURGERY & RECOVERY #1

On the eighth day after my hemorrhage and ultimate transfer to the Norfolk hospital for surgery, I was introduced to the doctor who would perform my coiling. *Coiling* is a term that both my husband and I were unfamiliar with, so meeting the doctor for the first time was comforting. The doctor was an interventional neuroradiologist who specialized in coiling. The timeframe allotted for discussion and introduction along with a decision to have the surgery was minimal, primarily because availabilities of physicians specializing in coiling were slim.

The doctor explained what would transpire, to what degree, the length of surgery, and the length of recovery, and he answered all questions my husband and I had. Within about half an hour from my time of arrival, I went in for surgery.

My surgery consisted of fixing the ruptured aneurysm, which was medically known as a pericallosal aneurysm, to minimize further danger. It was measured at four to five millimeters, and because the neck of this aneurysm was narrow, it was right for coiling. With three aneurysms, a lot of specialization and medical assessments were necessary to narrow down the culprit aneurysm. The aneurysm surgery was conducted under general anesthesia; I underwent a coil embolization, which consisted of a catheter being inserted through my groin and moved up to my brain to fill the aneurysm. I had one mild blood clot at the base of the aneurysm which was effectively treated during surgery.

I awoke from the surgery with all my motor skills functioning and quickly responded to the nurses. After the surgery, suture was used to secure the site on my groin, and I had to lie still in a specified position for about eight hours. With the expected pain, medication, IVs and follow-up care, I recovered through. A CT scan the following day showed that everything was functioning as projected.

While recovering in the neurosurgery intensive care unit, I was exposed to some wonderful nurses. They tended to my every need on schedule. Although I was cared for around the clock, the nights and early mornings seemed to warrant a lot more follow-up exams, checkups and other requirements.

My mother spent a few nights with me in the hospital. At seventy-four years old, she slept upright in chairs and frequently compromised her sleep to ensure I was still breathing; her presence was most reassuring.

Several days later I was discharged, given multiple medications, and told not to drive. When I arrived home, the problem I struggled with the most was being unable to walk. Because I had been bedridden for over thirteen days, it seemed as if my leg muscles had partially atrophied. My husband was very creative and became my physical therapist. With no formal training, he massaged me, applied heat to my body, and forced me to walk using his body as a crutch. The process was excruciating, and I eventually became mobile again.

THE WITNESSES' PERSPECTIVE

A few weeks later, I had the courage to visit the volleyball association where everything had occurred. I was concerned that I would be the topic of discussion (I thought people would say, "That's the player who passed out," "She's the one who almost died," etc.) and was also fearful of seeing the court where it had all happened.

Accounts from a few key people who had been there on the evening of the incident revealed the following stories. Their recollections indicated that I had backed up, tripped over my own feet, and then fallen onto my bottom. It also appeared that I was laughing for a minute, then I fell back all the way on the floor and my eyes rolled up in my head and I looked like I was having a seizure. Someone called the ambulance at that point, but in the meantime a few significant events occurred.

Apparently there were players with medical experience present, and some apparently realized I was chewing gum; they removed it and continued to watch over me. I was unresponsive for a moment.

I was told that a young lady named Gina from the opposing team got down to say a prayer for me, and she was joined by the referee and other players from my team. Shortly afterward, I regained consciousness and the ambulance arrived.

MY GUARDIAN

I was extremely curious to know who Gina was, and most importantly, I wanted to say thank you, because deep down I felt she had a lot to do with my still being alive. Several weeks later, while visiting the volleyball establishment, I made eye contact with someone walking toward me and smiling. I asked, "Are you Gina?" She said "Yes; it's so nice to see you. You look great."

We hugged like old friends who shared a bond. The ironic thing is that we had never officially met. We may have said hello in passing or shaken hands while playing against each other. I asked her to tell me everything as she remembered it. She was a member of the opposing team that evening. She witnessed everything that had transpired with one profound exception. She said that when I had passed out she felt an overwhelming and persistent pressure on her. The persistent pressure was that she needed to say a prayer for me. She said she fought the feeling continuously while asking why she should be the one to do this. She rationalized it and said, "Of all the people in the building, why should I say a prayer for her when I do not know her?" After struggling with her emotions for a while, she knelt down, touched my ankle, and started praying for me. Others joined her shortly thereafter.

She and I both broke down in tears when she told me the story. I was even more grateful to her than I had been, and I felt indebted to her. As she continued to share the experience with me, she also stated that her dad had died a couple of weeks after my incident, just before Christmas. I felt a great deal of sorrow for her, and we cried even more. I asked her what had happened to her dad, and she told me he had died of a massive brain aneurysm. I was so overwhelmed at that moment that I could not contain myself. Our conversation eventually ended with hugs, gratitude, and sorrow. I later struggled with the fact that there could have been a tradeoff— her dad's life for mine.

She also shared that her granddad had died of a brain aneurysm. As I became more knowledgeable of the condition, I encouraged her to have a magnetic resonance imagery (MRI) performed, because there appeared to be a family history.

SURGERY#2

My left aneurysm was diagnosed as a relatively broad-based six-millimeter MCA bifurcation aneurysm in my left internal carotid artery. Basically, it was the largest of the three and was not a candidate for coiling, so I would need to undergo my first craniotomy.

My procedure was to be conducted in another state by one of the best neurosurgeons available. The phrase used to describe this neurosurgeon was, "He has a reputation of performing miracles." Prior to my meeting him, I struggled with the thought of a craniotomy for weeks. The literature I read in a pamphlet and the pictures I saw on the internet describing what would happen were too vivid for me to deal with. The thought of my skull being opened was not easy to process. Having a side of my head shaved was the very least of my concerns.

I lost sleep, was afraid of being alone, was fearful of another rupture, and did not lift anything heavy. Simple body functions, such as bowel movements, sneezing, and coughing, were major fear factors that sometimes led to panic. I thought that anything too strenuous might cause a rupture and that I might not be as fortunate the second time around.

Throughout this period I noticed that I started suffering from hair loss on the back of my head. Each time I combed my hair, lots of hair came out in the comb and fell onto both my back and the ground. My family members looked at the sight and tried to console me. They said, "Don't worry about it" and refused to let me look at it. One day my curiosity got the best of me, and I took a small mirror, aligned it with the large one affixed to my bathroom wall, and took a look. What I saw was frightening, and the damage was grave. A hugh patch of hair was missing, and when I touched the area, more hair came out in my hand. I did not understand what was going on, because there was not an aneurysm near that area, nor was the hair loss subsiding. My imagination got the best of me and contributed further to my anxiety. I was eventually referred to a dermatologist. After explaining what my current medical condition was, the doctor told me that stress was the culprit. I had a huge bald spot on the back of my head. Because of everything I was enduring, the thought of imminent death became prominent in my mind. I did gain the courage to minimize that thought.

On the morning of the procedure, I was to be the first patient for my doctor. I was wheeled into a room for preparation, paperwork, and sedation, and after some time passed, I was told that I had been bumped. Another patient's situation was more urgent than mine. I was relieved that I had more time to just relax and talk with my husband. My thoughts did, however, go out to the patient who preceded me. While watching the news on television, I heard that Christopher Reeve's wife had passed away from her lung cancer.

I compared her to me, saying, "she never smoked and I never participated in anything that could have caused my aneurysms." It certainly wasn't right!

As my turn neared, I was told that they were almost finished with the other patient and that they were turning the equipment around. The lady who preceded me had had her surgery on the side of her head opposite the side mine was to be on. At that point I knew my blood pressure was spiraling out of control. I visualized every possible outcome, and I experienced a multitude of emotions. I eventually gave in to this, broke down, and cried like a child. Once I had been taken to the preparation room and given some medication, I composed myself and chose to visualize a positive outcome before I was anesthetized. When I later regained consciousness, I felt good and had apparently already passed all the necessary verbal tests, though I had no recollection of doing so.

RECOVERY

I was cared for very well in the hospital, and as expected, I slept a lot. I was taken to my room, where I realized I had a roommate for the first time. I later found out that my roommate had had the same surgery I did, however, hers had been performed on the opposite side of her head. I was surprised when I realized she was the lady who had preceded me on the morning of my surgery. Although we did not have in-depth conversations, probably because we were both recovering from the trauma of having brain surgery, we were casually appreciative of each other's company and had solace in knowing that we had both experienced the same thing and survived.

The surgical site was stapled with about forty staples from the center of my head down to my left ear. I was sporting a very bad semimohawk due to my head being shaved on one side and bald in the back. Additionally, I had some new hardware implanted— titanium pins and screws. I also had a drainage tube in the back of my head which was to be removed within a few days.

My doctor indicated that the artery walls of my aneurysm looked so weak that he anticipated it would have ruptured within a week to a month. With time on my hands, I wondered if I would be setting off metal detectors more now than before, or if water would seep into my brain when I washed my hair or swam. After a short stay, my roommate was discharged, and I followed a day later.

My recovery at home was not bad. As a matter of fact, I healed rather quickly. I was on so many medications that I felt like a walking pharmacy. My pain medication was extremely helpful, and within a few weeks, I no longer needed them continuously. I had previously asked my doctor if jumping would make my new head hardware shift, and he had gently smiled and said no. I was creative with my headgear, because I didn't want to scare others by exposing them to my multiple staples.

My discharge orders involved returning for the removal of my staples within a certain timeframe. I envisioned lying on a comfortable bed and being given local anesthesia prior to the removal of my staples. The reality was vastly different. Upon meeting my nurse, I asked about the kind of medication I would receive. She said I wouldn't be given any medication while the staples were being removed. I said, "You're kidding, right?" She smiled and said, "No, but I will use a very small instrument." When I saw it, I said, "Is that a staple remover?" and she said, "Basically, yes."

I tried to relax as much as possible on the table, and my husband held my hand tightly. The first and second staples removed were not too bad. By the time we reached the fifth one, I was grabbing her arm. I said, "We need to take a break." She was pleasantly patient and supportive, and she told me to let her know when I was ready to continue. After about five minutes, I reluctantly said I was ready again. She suggested we start from a different part of my head, and I agreed. The succession continued, and I squealed, moaned, and groaned because some of staples were embedded a little deeper than others. I am sure she took some skin with some of the staples. The struggle continued with many pauses in between and me asking, "Is it finished yet?" The torment ended with all of us laughing at the experience.

Over the weeks that followed, feeling my brain heal was unsettling. I felt circular headaches, shooting headaches, and a barrage of unfamiliar events near my temple. Although most of the occurrences did not warrant medication in the later weeks, the condition was nerve wracking. In spite of what the doctor said regarding my progression, I continued on an emotional rollercoaster, wondering if the surgery really worked, if something else was growing, if they had forgotten to put something back in place, etc. Those emotional concerns were more aggravating than the surgery itself. My fear of being left alone was also heightened. Although I knew that the two aneurysms that had posed the greatest risks had been taken care of, the new physical changes in my head, coupled with the unresolved aneurysm and my emotional torment, continued my discontent.

SURGERY#3

As time passed, I had some great days, while other days were a little challenging. I tired easily, was a little forgetful, repeated things, and continued to struggle with my emotions. Planning what was to be my final procedure was important. I felt it would help to alleviate my fears and bring some normalcy back into my life. Although the final aneurysm was the smallest, I did not underestimate it, and I looked forward to having it coiled. Because I had experienced a coiling before, I knew this would be less intrusive to my head. The third aneurysm was described as "A right middle cerebral fiburcation measuring about 3 to 3.5 mm with a small neck."

An appointment was made for my third and final procedure, and I had mixed emotions about it. Finally, I would have some closure and a coiling instead of a craniotomy. On the morning of my procedure, my doctor indicated that he thought the coiling of that aneurysm might be challenging based on its shape; he told me that he had stated that in an earlier visit, but I had forgotten. He said he would examine it and if he thought it might cause more harm than good, he would not undertake the procedure. I did not want to hear that, but I hoped for the best. I was put to sleep, and it seemed like I was awakened within a half an hour. In my moment of fog, there was a lot of discussion, and many people were tending to me. The only thing I wanted to hear was that the coiling had been completed.

My doctor arrived, and the news was not what I anticipated. He said my aneurysm wasn't coilable and that I would have to undergo another craniotomy. I was heartbroken, disappointed, and scared. The craniotomy was scheduled for a few days later. The emotional torture was hard to bear in spite of my husband's efforts to keep me occupied and happy.

The morning of my final procedure arrived, and I approached it with mixed emotions. Yes, I was glad it would finally be over, but I also did not look forward to another craniotomy. I was fully alert and awake when I was taken into the surgical room. The nurses and doctors introduced themselves and did their part to make me comfortable. I looked at all the equipment above me and wondered what equipment would be used to open my skull. I said a prayer, as I had done prior to the other surgeries, and started feeling very relaxed. That's all I remembered until I was awakened later. The procedure had been executed without complications.

When I looked in the mirror for the first time, I almost didn't recognize myself. I had a scar similar to the one left by my first craniomity, but this one was on the right side of my head. My face was extensively swollen, the right side of my head was shaved, and I was once again sporting multiple staples. My eldest brother, whom I'm extremely close with, came to visit me in the hospital, and after looking at me all swollen and stapled, he broke down in tears. He and I had transitioned through and achieved multiple evolutions, and I had never once seen him cry. I didn't know he possessed tears until this moment.

My mobility was improved at my own pace. My doctor recommended frequent walks as I could tolerate them. With my husband by my side and serving as my crutch, I made progress in small amounts. One evening, while walking in the hospital arm-in-arm with my husband, I suddenly broke out in a cold sweat and passed out. That moment was a complete mystery to me. My husband was the one who told me that I had blacked out. My condition was probably a mini seizure. Subsequently, I was discharged.

At home I tried to normalize my life as much as possible. Within a couple of weeks, I started to take walks in the neighborhood with my husband, then with my cell phone, and eventually on my own. I progressed to going to the gym and riding the elliptical machine or the stationary bike. I did not lift weights, because in my mind the possibility still existed that I could strain something, or worse, cause another aneurysm to grow, even though I knew neither aerobic exercise nor weightlifting contributed to my condition. I also realized weeks later that I was able to be left alone. The first instances of my being home alone involved me staying on the sofa and keeping the phone next to me as if it were my security. I also refrained from going upstairs and showering when left alone.

I felt a need to visit the optometrist, because my eyes were extra sensitive to light. I noticed that when in an automobile at dusk, the headlights from oncoming vehicles were piercing to my eyes. I would often blink, look away, or close my eyes. My vision was clear, but slightly peculiar. My examination indicated that my vision was normal; however, my optic nerve was swollen. That was another revelation. Once I explained my recent surgeries to the optometrist, she referred me to an ophthalmologist.

The ophthalmologist conducted a barrage of examinations, many of which I had never encountered before. My favorite—and I use the term sparingly—was the peripheral screening exam. With one eye covered, I had to look at a screen, and whenever I saw a minute speck of light, I had to press a buzzer. That examination had me thinking I was seeing things. I thought it was worse than taking a hearing exam. That process was ongoing, and I continually passed the screening examinations, but my optic nerve remained swollen.

My swollen optic nerve, coupled with the fact that I started experiencing some difficulties with consistent minor headaches, led to some troubleshooting of the symptoms. It was recommended that I undergo a lumbar puncture, otherwise known as a spinal tap, to see if I was experiencing swelling of my brain. When the process was explained to me I said, "Not again, I cannot take another hospital stay and certainly don't have any room on my body for more injections and needles." Fortunately, the process only took one day, but the experience was unforgettable. I was once again admitted to the hospital. I was injected in my back near my spine a few times to numb the area, and then I had to bend over a table, holding it tightly while others held me in place. After a few injections, spinal fluid was withdrawn and tested. The results were favorable, and I had to lie in a designated position for several hours to prevent a potentially major headache. I was extremely obedient.

While at home one day, my husband offered to shave my head completely. In spite of the fact that my hair looked really jagged, I resisted submitting to the bald look. I eventually gave in, and my husband shaved my head completely bald. I thought it looked rather cute.

THE UNEXPECTED HAPPENED

I had finally regained my confidence and independence. I was comfortable alone and able to drive, and so I returned to work. I was twelve days short of six months since my final of three surgeries, and I felt I was well on my way to full recovery. I no longer had a fear of participating in anything that required jumping, but I was cautious.

One night something unexpected happened! On September 28, 2006, I turned in for bed like I normally do. The day's events were normal, and my health was continuously improving. I was awakened sometime after 2:00 a.m. by a desire to urinate, and I realized I was in different surroundings. My daughter and husband were present, and I was wearing a hospital gown. "What happened and where am I?" I asked. I was told that I had experienced a grand mal seizure and had been taken to the hospital via ambulance. I had no recollection of the event, not even a small memory. I was eventually discharged and told that I was not allowed to drive for six months.

My husband later filled me in on the events of the night. He told me that during the night, I hit him several times, but he thought I was telling him that he was snoring. Because the hitting was continual and strong, and because I did not speak to him, which was out of the norm, he realized something was wrong and turned the light on. To his surprise, I was having a seizure. He said I was rigid, frothing at the mouth, and clamping my teeth down with a vengeance. He also stated that my breathing was very sharp and deep. He checked my vital signs, turned me on my side, and called the ambulance while he continued to monitor my movements. All appeared normal for a person having a seizure until my shallow breathing stopped. He said that was the most fearful he had ever been throughout my ordeal, but he kept his composure. He checked for breathing by putting his hand on my chest and noticed that his hand raised and lowered. Then he checked for my pulse and found it. From that point on, it was just a matter of waiting for the ambulance. The ambulance arrived, confirmed that I had experienced a seizure and that all my bodily functions were operating properly.

Prior to that incident, I had never had a seizure, and I still don't know what the symptoms are. I followed up with a neurologist who conducted an EEG (brain scan) on me. She told me that there was a lot of activity going on in my head. I was placed on antiseizure medication for six months and once again restricted from driving. The entire episode reevoked my fears of loneliness, death, etc. A new fear also emerged: I feared going to sleep. My first few nights of going to bed after the seizure were filled with anxiety, but I had to sleep. When I awoke the following mornings, I was very grateful and thanked the Lord. Future EEGs showed positive changes, but it was recommended that I remain on the medication for one year as a precaution. Follow-up care and tests would dictate if I needed the medication for life. I resumed work with the assistance of my coworkers. They created a plan to transport me back and forth to work.

SYMBOLISMS

1. The night my aneurysm ruptured, I was in a room filled with many people. It could have ruptured while driving on the way to or from the organization.

2. From a standing position, and despite my being six feet two inches tall, I fell on my bottom and then fell back on the floor instead of falling directly to the floor.

3. People with whom I previously had only casual communication with (volleyball opponents and teammates) prayed for me and did what they could to sustain me until the ambulance arrived.

4. On the way to the hospital, the voice that said, "Oh, she is a Senior Chief; well, I'm a Chief, so she is in good hands" was heaven sent.

5. My husband was not out of town.

6. After arriving in the intensive care unit, two of my nurses turned out to be from my native country. Throughout the course of my stay, one braided my hair and one became my sounding board. They both extended prayers and assured me that I would be okay.

7. I was placed in all the right hands and tended to by the best doctors and nurses in their respective fields. One of my nurses from the Norfolk hospital was extremely kind; she went above and beyond to ensure all my needs were met. I will be forever grateful to her.

8. My sister and brother-in-law, who were visiting for the first time over the Thanksgiving holiday, extended their stay to accommodate my family and me.

9. When my driving was restricted, my husband was able to modify his work schedule to accommodate me.

10. Someone told me it wasn't my time.

PHOTOS

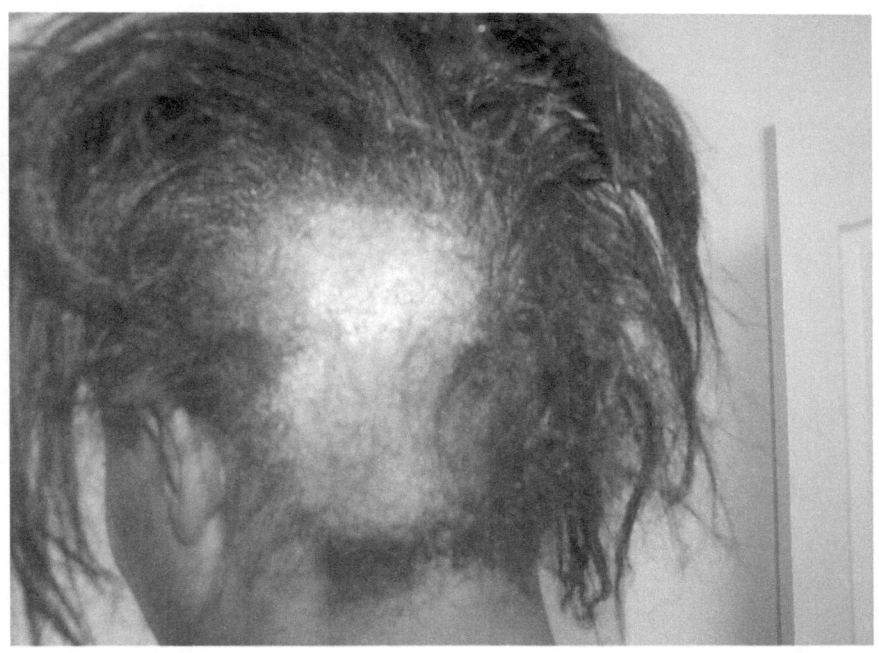

Hair loss due to excess stress

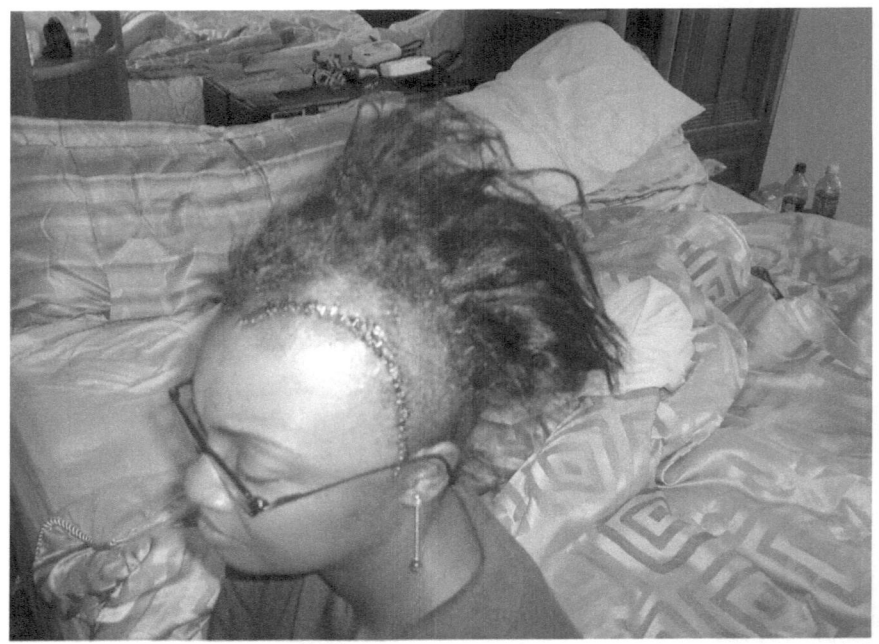

My first craniotomy

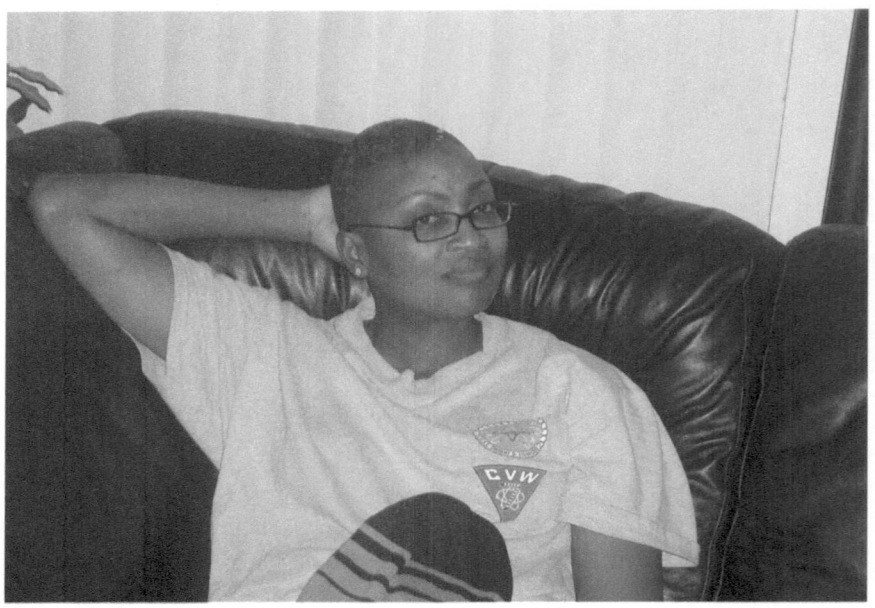

Embracing my new look after two craniotomies

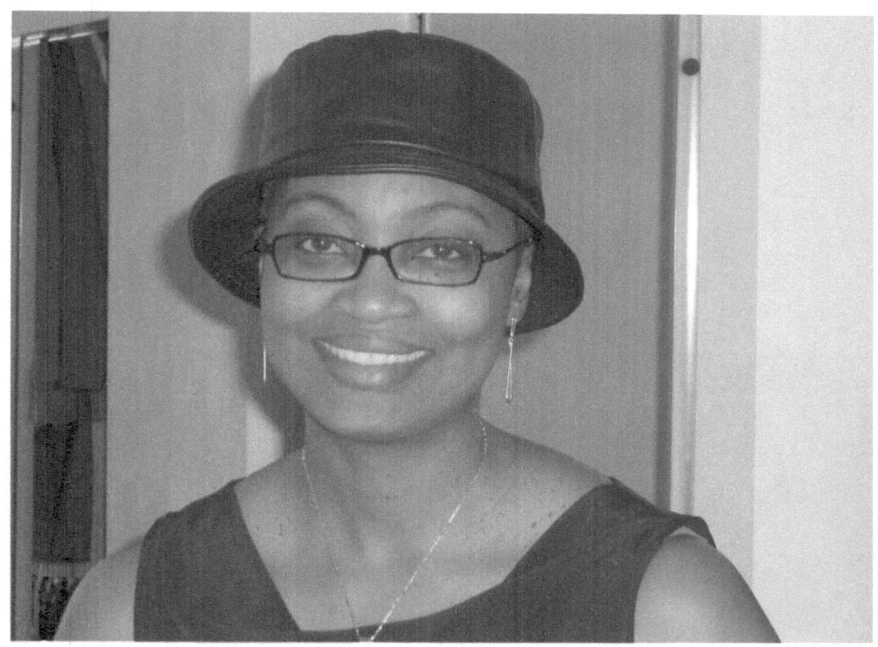

Optimism in spite of the circumstances

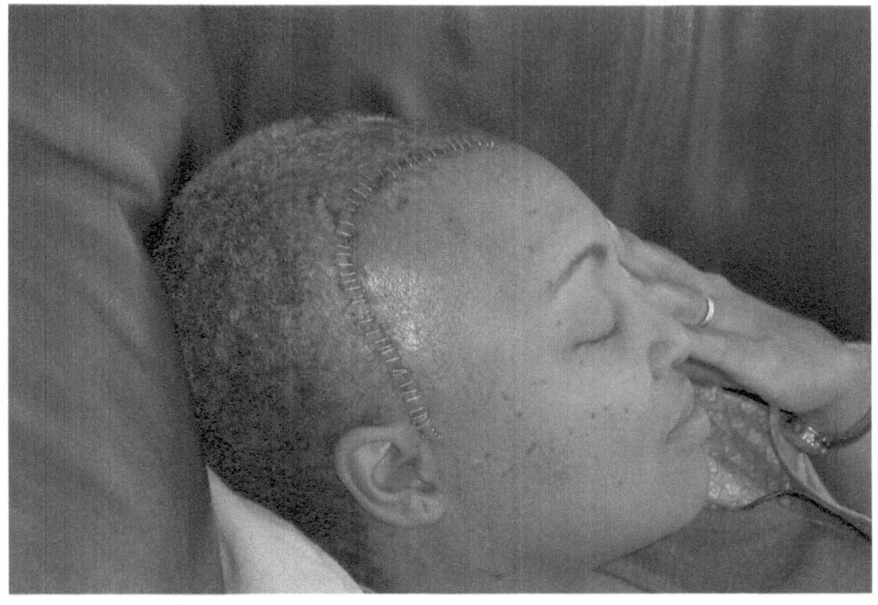

Recovering from the second craniotomy

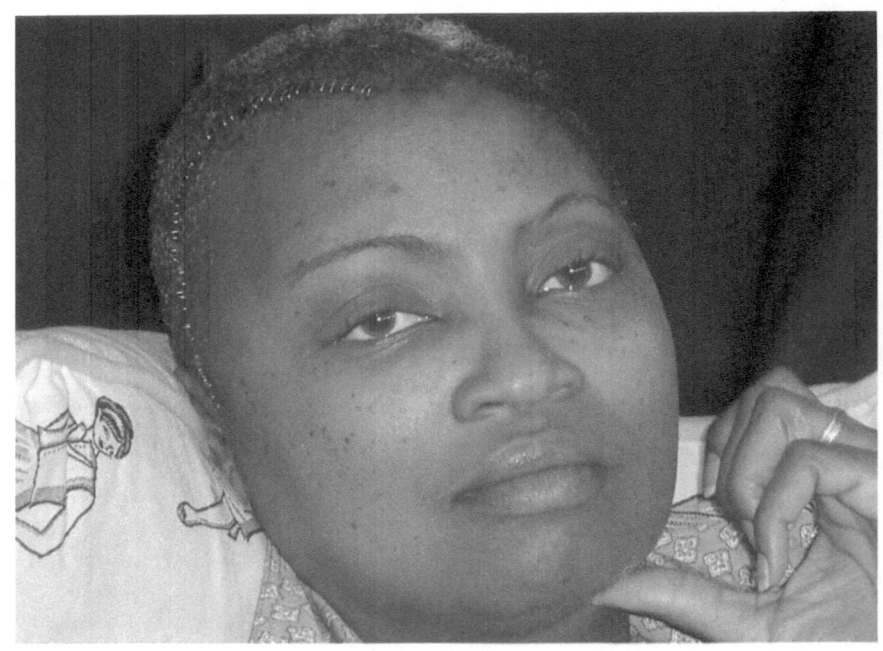

My eyes say it all!

AWARENESS & THE FUTURE

My three surgeries occurred at six-week intervals. I wanted to get them over with as soon as medically possible. Throughout the process, the psychological changes were unbearable. My support system helped to maintain my sanity. I had visions of myself lying in a circle of prayers, and that vision started at the onset of my hospital stay. I was lying down, and people around me were continuously praying. I believe the prayers extended to me by family, friends, and coworkers materialized into my vision and contributed to my miraculous survival.

The phones never stopped ringing, and everyone I spoke to either started or ended the conversation with a religious statement. I was extremely grateful and realized that I had not placed enough emphasis on attending church and serving God as I should have. That is one area I vowed to work on as soon as I was able.

A combination of stories I had heard of people dying from aneurysms and my own personal experience compounded my anxieties and heightened my cautiousness. Living with an untreated aneurysm or two was also a daily reminder that I was still ill, regardless of how I looked or felt at the time. The doctors were unable to give me guarantees regarding whether or not my aneurysms would rupture while I was awaiting surgery. I came to the conclusion that I was living with time bombs inside my head and that time was my enemy. The fear of dying was real, but my willingness to live was stronger. Inner strength, belief, trust, and—most importantly—hope paved the way for my endurance and mental stability. Now imagine someone facing this situation without hope or support.

Brain aneurysms are sneaking up on many people, and by the time they reveal their presence, it's often too late for many. Victims of this deadly disease have a 50 percent chance of survival after a rupture. The universal knowledge about high blood pressure, cholesterol, various cancers, etc. is widespread and addressed in most medical settings and on questionnaires.

No one talks about aneurysms; however, when a discussion ensues on the topic, everyone seems to know someone who passed away from or survived an aneurysm. Aneurysms form in many areas of the body, and the consequences of an aneurism can be very brutal. The understanding of how one gets a brain aneurysm is still sketchy. The best explanation I have heard thus far is "You were probably born with it." I have no family history of the disease.

The catastrophe of aneurysm rupture is so prevalent and life changing that more research and publicity is necessary. It should probably be incorporated in medical checkups and moved to the forefront of major illnesses. The symptoms associated with the disease are not present in many of its victims; all too often, it comes as a surprise. Many pamphlets show pictures of the elderly, indicating they are the major group of people afflicted with the disease, but I was only 42 years old and have heard of younger people including teenagers having aneurysms. The symptoms predicated, such as high blood pressure, migraines, and head trauma, are also not consistent for the masses and can be very misleading.

There is still a lot I don't understand about aneurysms. I do know that I will be placed on a specified cycle to have MRIs completed for the rest of my life to ensure there is no new aneurysm growth.

To all the survivors of aneurysms—to those who have gone on and to those who are walking around unaware of their condition—I empathize completely.